# IS AN
# ALLERGY
# TO FOOD
## SPOILING
## YOUR LIFE?

Keith Scott-Mumby MD, MB ChB, HMD, PhD

**Is An Allergy To Food Spoiling Your Life?**
by Keith Scott-Mumby, MD
Copyright © 2012-2018 Keith Scott-Mumby, MD

ISBN: 978-0-9913188-6-5
Published by Mother Whale Inc.
PO Box 19452, Reno, Nevada, 89511, USA

**Publisher Disclaimer**
This book is intended as a reference volume only, not as a medical manual. The ideas, procedures and suggestions contained herein are not intended as a substitute for consulting with your personal medical practitioner.

Neither the publisher nor the author shall be liable for any loss or damage allegedly arising from any information or suggestions in this book, howsoever applied or misapplied. Further, if you have a medical problem, we urge you to seek advice from a licensed medical practitioner.

# AN IMPORTANT NOTE FROM THE AUTHOR

Please do not pass any word you don't fully understand in context, without looking up its' meaning.

This seems a simple thing to ask, but many people are lazy in this respect and would prefer to try and guess the meaning of a word. There is a (very slight) chance of guessing correctly this way, true.

However, it's important to understand that, even if the meaning is guessed correctly, the mind remains troubled by the word, because it is inherently not understood.

*It works as if you have no real meaning for it.*

Why is that important?

Because, as English science fiction writer H G Wells tells us: "Every word of which a man is ignorant represents an idea of which he is ignorant." [These days, of course, one must say man or woman.]

In other words, you won't *fully understand* what you are reading. You won't fully "get it." That results in steadily increasing alienation from the text.

In this case, it means missing out on fabulously valuable ideas that are assembled in this TOOLBOOK, with the power to change your life.

Failure may not happen straight away, but it WILL happen, for sure. It's very important to realize that just one word that is not grasped may be enough to derail you completely, many pages or chapters later. Tiny becomes HUGE!

It's a bit like a thorn or a splinter that gets into a person's skin. It may not seem much at the time but three weeks later, the person has life-threatening gangrene and may have to have a limb amputated.

From a seemingly inconsequential beginning there can be a fatal result. In the case of study this may mean the person doesn't grasp the materials at all – or, even worse, just gives up – because he or she basically "lost it" early on.

These days it's easy to check the meaning of words, using one or more online dictionary:

- www.dictionary.com

- www.freeonlinedictionary.com

- www.merriam-webster.com

- www.collinsdictionary.com

To name just a few. You don't need a huge dictionary by your side these days; just your cell phone and an internet connection!

Simply type in the search string "[WORD] definition" (for example, *internecine definition*) and several reputable sites will instantly appear.

Thank you for your attention to this important study detail!

# CONTENTS

# INTRODUCTION

A doctor friend of mine who regarded himself to be in perfect health, did some experimental testing on himself to discover whether he had any food allergies.

He uncovered an allergy to wheat and as a further test, he omitted wheat from his diet.

To his surprise, he no longer felt tired at the end of a busy day and woke in the morning with a feeling of exhilaration instead of his usual dread of a heavy day's work. The doctor suddenly realized that his perfect health was far from being as good as it could be.

When bread, which is usually regarded as the staff of life, disagrees with you, and you are an unsuspecting victim of what is happening consequently, you can come to regard health as a mere absence of disease.

A positive sense of well-being with plenty of energy always ready for use is what should be regarded as normal health.

An allergy to the food you are eating everyday can take the edge off your enjoyment of life, can cause you to feel under the weather without anything definite to complain about, or can actually be the cause of severe inexplicable illness.

# SECTION 1:
# THE UNSUSPECTED ENEMY

Food allergy has been well described as the unsuspected enemy. Because this source of illness tends to remain unsuspected, it is a pleasant surprise to discover how easy it can be to get well, once the possibility of food allergy is taken into consideration.

It is usual to think of food allergy in terms of the type of illness which results from an allergy to strawberries or to shellfish. These foods however are not eaten on a day to day basis, and the violence of the reaction leaves little opportunity for the source of the illness to remain unsuspected. There is a marked reaction to the food, which dies down and disappears within a short time.

But there is an entirely different clinical picture when the food to which you are allergic is a staple item of your diet that you eat every day of your life, perhaps several times each day.

Under these circumstances, the body adapts to the allergic process and the reaction disappears to become a masked allergy. This adaptation of the body may last a lifetime or may become exhausted at any time under stress.

When the adaptation by the body is complete there are no symptoms, but if the strain of coping with the allergy wears down the adaptive process then a whole variety of symptoms may break surface.

At different times in a person's life these breakthrough manifestations of the underlying masked allergy, may present themselves in a wide variety of illnesses.

## Changing Pattern in Life

Let us take a typical life story of a person who is allergic to cow's milk. If bottle-fed as a baby, there are considerable feeding difficulties. Baby gets a lot of wind and mother gets many sleepless nights.

There may be a long period with a runny nose, repeated ear troubles, sore throats, constant colds and tonsils and adenoids get removed. The adaptive process may become complete from time to time and all symptoms may disappear.

The allergic patient may enjoy periods of excellent health when nothing appears to be wrong. But it is quite usual for the patient to have growing pains, to be over or under active, to have learning difficulties, troublesome headaches, be highly susceptible to infections and suffer frequent colds and 'flu attacks.

At puberty the patient's story may take a dramatic turn, all symptoms may disappear completely, or everything may get worse. When puberty brings trouble, it can come in many forms; migraine, asthma, eczema, acne, depression, behavior problems even vandalism can suddenly turn on as a result of the masked allergy becoming partially unmasked.

In girls, all manner of menstrual problems may be a result of an unsuspected allergy to foods or chemicals. It seems as though the body becomes supersensitive to its own hormones and any variation in the hormone balance occurring at puberty, at menstruation, during pregnancy or at the menopause may all cause symptoms of varying degrees.

These symptoms may be premenstrual tension, heavy painful periods, absence of periods, sickness in pregnancy, toxemia of pregnancy, depression after confinement and all those unpleasant symptoms commonly associated with change of life.

One of the main characteristics of illness due to food allergy is the wide variety of symptoms.

Any bodily system can be upset by food allergy and in any one patient one or more systems can be involved. The system involved can change from one period of life to another.

A child with eczema, moves on to asthma, grows out of asthma and develops stomach ulcers or the irritable bowel syndrome. Stress helps to exhaust the adaptive process of the body and aggravate the symptoms. In this manner, it often appears as though stress is the cause of the trouble. The patient may have to endure psychotherapy and when this fails to cure the trouble, drugs may be used to suppress the symptoms.

An allergy to food and chemicals seems to guarantee an adverse reaction to drugs and medicines, the patient tends to get worse and becomes a very difficult case, ending up allergic to almost everything.

## Woolly Brain Syndrome

In a typical case of masked food allergy, the patient may suffer mainly from involvement of the central nervous system. Perhaps the most distressing symptom of all is what has been described by patients as the woolly brain syndrome.

An inability to concentrate, a confusion of thinking, an impairment of memory and a tendency to just sit in an inactive torpor, are all symptoms which cause great distress to a patient who is normally highly intelligent, very industrious, and exceptionally competent.

Depression is a common and distressing symptom. I have often heard patients with this complaint say that they would kill themselves if they could only bring themselves to do it. Life becomes intolerable.

This state of affairs can put an impossible strain on a marriage. In this condition the person does not wish to be touched and may turn nasty in response to any sort of advance from the marital partner.

These patients often come to be labelled neurotic hypochondriacs and because they cannot explain or understand their own predicament they often come to believe themselves to be insane or going insane.

Once these patients are put on drugs and become addicted to drugs the true situation is virtually impossible to untangle and many must be ending their days in mental hospitals.

## Becoming an Epidemic

This whole problem of unsuspected allergy seems to be on the increase. No research has been done in this area and we have no factual data to establish the prevalence of this condition nor its cause.

Nevertheless, a great deal of circumstantial evidence is available from the histories of patients with proven masked allergies.

It is usual to discover that some-thing other than the mother's colostrum was the first material to enter the stomach after birth. The onset of symptoms is very often triggered by medical treatment. Patients very often recover when additives and pollutants are carefully eliminated from their food and drink.

It would seem that an epidemic of allergic disease has been started by failure of breast feeding, by pollution of the environment, by the addition of chemicals to our food, air, and water and to the injudicious use of drugs and medicines.

These are enormous problems to be faced in tackling the illnesses caused by this unsuspected enemy, but those problems are miniscule compared to the problems created by ignorance of the phenomenon of food allergy. The first step is to unmask the enemy and then it will be possible to assess the full extent of the problem.

The door will open to the elimination of much illness and to the creation of better health.

# SECTION 2:
# THE BRAIN AS A
# TARGET ORGAN

The number one target or what we call a shock organ, which gets hit in almost every case, is the brain and the results of this can be incredibly complex and fascinating.

Many universal symptoms are often a result; fatigue being the outstanding one. The fiery food or pathogen excites the brain, which goes into overdrive and then soon packs up exhausted.

Thus, revving your grey matter with caffeine all day is a pretty dumb act; it will lead to nervous exhaustion, which then requires more caffeine to get it firing again, and so on, round and round in a vicious cycle.

Quite apart from brain stimulation or fatigue, other symptoms can take on an incredible shifting variety of patterns. The brain is the organ which summates our principal sensations and interprets them.

Any toxic overload can lead to hallucinations, excitation, mania, and hyper activity; the reverse, which often follows quickly, leads downwards, through increasing fatigue, inertia, depression, slowing down and finally coma.

I've seen allergies (food and environmental) lead to heightened sexual feelings, murderous assault, schizophrenic psychosis, woolly thinking, hallucination, hyperactivity, depression, anxiety, learning difficulties, dyslexia, and autism spectrum disorder.

## Protean and Bizarre

The truth is that brain overdrive or fatigue states can lead to hundreds of symptoms, if not thousands.

Some of these are protean, bizarre, variable, and subjective (doctors don't like the word subjective in this context: if only one patient gets it, they react with suspicion that this cannot be a real symptom)!

But really, if the patient were to imagine things, is that too not just another symptom? I mean, duh!

Examples of such bizarre and subjective responses I have seen over the years include things like "hot water running down the inside of my skin," "feeling like I am seeing the world down a long, dark tube" and "feeling dirty and wanting to strip my clothes off."

Protean is just an old-fashioned word that means changeable; like the mythic figure of the Greek sea-god Proteus. He would appear in many different forms, such as a man, a beast, a seductive siren, and so on.

In this case, the patient would visit the doctor one week with headaches; next week it would be diarrhea or colic; the week after, nightmares and hallucinations; a month later excessive fluid retention. So, the doctor would inevitably label such patients as hypochondriac and symptoms therefore "all in the mind."

But somatic reactions too can be subjective. I have had many patients whose epilepsy traced to brain excitation from fiery allergy foods. Not too surprising, except that nobody else seemed to recognize it!

# SECTION 3:
# TAKE A PERSONAL
# INVENTORY

You can get a better appreciation of whether a food allergy may be spoiling your life by reading the following list of (just some) health conditions that can and will respond very well to the food allergy approach.

## Conditions Often Rooted in Food Allergies

- Asthma
- Eczema
- Urticaria (hives)
- Rhinitis (seasonal and perennial)
- Catarrh and sinusitis
- Gas, flatulence
- Abdominal bloating
- Arthritis (all types but especially rheumatoid)
- Lack of energy and ambition
- Inability to think clearly (foggy brain or "woolly" brain)
- Behavioral disorders in children
- Dizziness
- Panic attacks
- ADD, ADHD
- Autism
- Learning disorders
- Colitis and Crohn's disease

- Eating disorders (anorexia and bulimia)
- Diarrhea
- Constipation
- Hemorrhoids
- Headaches
- Hypertension
- Mastitis or breast pains
- Meniere's disease
- Migraine
- Mouth ulcers
- Multiple Sclerosis
- Myalgic encephalo-myelitis or Fibromyalgia
- Polymyalgia
- Pre-menstrual tension
- Psoriasis
- Recurring Cystitis
- Alcoholism
- Anxiety
- Depression
- Violent behavior, smashing up attacks
- Frigidity
- Hypothyroidism
- Impotence
- Nephrotic syndrome
- Schizophrenia
- Depression
- Alzheimer's disease
- Parkinson's disease
- Cardiac arrhythmias (especially tachycardia)
- Angina
- High moods

- Low moods
- Variable moods
- Hypertension
- Overweight
- Underweight
- Variable weight
- Hyperhidrosis (excessive sweating, not related to exercise)
- Abnormal fatigue, not helped by rest
- Diabetes (both types but especially type II)

[With acknowledgements to Theron Randolph, Richard Mackarness, Vicky Rippere, and Marshall Mandell.]

That's not to say all these conditions are wholly, 100%, caused by "fire in the belly" (though some are).

But as I said, the influence of the extreme high level of intestinal inflammation that is present in humans today is such that, once it is corrected, many of the more serious conditions will regress or, quite often, disappear altogether.

## Other Disease Models

I don't want you to misunderstand a list like this and how it works. These are really symptoms and diseases related to a body in overload; that is, stressed outside a comfortable, working physiological and metabolic range.

Not one of the conditions from this list is concretely indicative of a food or chemical allergy, or any other cause of inflammation.

So, it would be wrong to light on, say, an eating disorder, overweight or depression and say that must be caused by a food allergy or intolerance.

It's really about quantity. The truth is that the more items from this list you suffer from, the more likely it is to be an overload of the kind I'm writing about.

One or two items would be suggestive; five, six or seven, make it probable. A person with a skin rash and fatigue, with occasional bouts of abdominal bloating and diarrhea, I would say, very likely has "fire in the belly" and would be well advised to check out the possibility, using the methods I give in this book.

It's also about appropriateness. If someone was depressed and lethargic, with no real reason; for example, he or she had a good life, without lack of material goods and has a loving partner or spouse, it's worth checking this out. Many a marriage has been saved by following the route I lay out in this book.

Neither is this meant to exclude other working health models. For example, many practitioners who know their stuff (I mean really know their stuff), when confronted with eczema would think of a "hot liver"; a Chinese traditional medicine specialist would think of too much Yang or deficiencies in the lung and kidney systems; a classically-trained homeopath would certainly think of a sulfur constitution; and a good counselor would ask about stress.

Using a treatment modality from these other models might also produce a good result. That would not make it unlikely that "fire in the belly" was present.

Over forty years as a clinician, I can tell you that disease always has multiple causative components, never just one trigger. Food and bowel inflammations are one of the commonest of all contributive factors to a whole host of diseases and mental states.

# SECTION 4:
# WHAT YOU CAN DO TO
# CLEAR THE PROBLEM

The best part of this is that you can usually clear the problems entirely, by experimenting with what you eat. You don't need a doctor and medicines are not required; in fact, chemicals, such as medicines, may make things worse for a person who is sensitive.

This is not to say that everything is a food allergy.

But diet adjustments are a great place to start because there is usually some kind of beneficial result and they are relatively easy to do. If you can feel much better just avoiding, say, milk or wheat, that is far easier than battling against multiple environmental shocks and stressors.

The reason is simple if you understand the overload principle: avoiding one stressor, especially if it is an important one, may free your body defenses up enough so that it can cope with the rest, without your help!

## Symptoms of Food Addictions

Some patients are amazed to realize that food allergies often cause addictions; in fact, a person can become dependent on one or more foods to relieve their symptoms.

That seems strange, till you think of heroin addiction: yes, the heroin relives the unpleasant withdrawal symptoms—but only because it is causing them in the first place!

Well, it works the same way with food. So, beware if you give in to food binges or food cravings!

Other symptoms that strongly suggest food addiction are:
- Feeling unwell when skipping a meal (withdrawal symptoms)
- Slow getting started in the morning
- Feeling tired, crabby, or unwell on waking (also a sign of food addiction)

The last may seem strange: most everybody wakes up feeling bad, don't they? True, but as I have been teaching for decades, that's because almost everyone is suffering the addiction effects of allergy.

Think about this: by the time we wake in the morning, we may not have eaten for 10- 14 hours; that's more than enough time to set up withdrawal symptoms. With breakfast, we get our first "fix" of wheat, sugar, caffeine, or whatever and the symptoms start to clear right away.

You don't believe me? Wait until you have followed the instruction in this section and you'll see the amazing truth of what I say.

For more in this phenomenon and extra detail and help on exploring the subject of allergy and intolerance foods, you can't do better than get yourself a full copy of my best-selling book Diet Wise. It will more than repay the study. There's more information about it at the back of this booklet.

Meantime, the following sections will give you a basic program to work with.

# SECTION 5:
# THE SECRET OF FOOD
# ALLERGY TEST DIETING

The secret of successful identification of food allergies is to give up sufficient foods to be able to feel well, then to re-introduce these foods one at a time, so that detecting a reaction is relatively easy. We call this elimination and challenge dieting.

It rarely works to give up just one food at a time because anyone who is ill is almost certain to have more than one allergy. If it was simply one major allergen, the person would have spotted it eventually, as indeed some lucky people do.

Dr. Doris Rapp of New York coined an instructive term: the "eight nails in the shoe trap". She points out that if you have eight nails sticking out in your shoe, and then pull just one of these nails, you will still not be comfortable – because of the other seven. It can be the same with multiple allergies. You must work at it just that little bit harder.

Make no mistake, elimination diets can be tough; they should be. But it is important to remember that I am talking here of a trial diet—an experimental procedure you would carry out for a couple of weeks or so. You do not need to stay on a tough diet long-term; indeed, you are specifically cautioned not to do so, otherwise you run into problems caused by inadequate nutritional sources.

The purpose of the strict "test" diet is to isolate the culprits. Once you know these, you can eat most anything else. This means you shift into a maintenance diet, solely avoiding these offending foods, something you stay on for months or years.

Almost anyone who feels much better by avoiding one or two foods has the will power to continue; the rewards are high! Please don't mix up these two grades of diet. You'll suffer needlessly.

## Three-Tiered Inflammatory Food Elimination and Identification

The rest of this section is given over to discussing three-tiered dieting, from which you can choose the most appropriate approach for you or your family.

In following the instructions, it is vital that in all cases you also avoid manufactured foods. This is not because food additives are a common intolerance problem (they are surprisingly uncommon, in fact) but because manufactured foods contain numerous foodstuffs that are hidden and disguised, such as corn starch, wheat, sugar, egg and other notable allergens.

Don't trust the labeling, it may be misleading and throw the whole test. Just eat only fresh whole versions of the foods allowed, in other words nothing from tins, packets, bottles and jars.

Don't even trust to foods cooked and packages by supermarkets and stores. It may cost you the results you are looking for.

Special note: people often ask me about using organic foods in an elimination diet. The answer is yes, it is always better to eat organic, if you can. But that may not be easy, and it is not really necessary. Almost everyone will feel better by eating ordinary commercial food supplies, providing they are fresh.

Only if you are very sensitive or very poorly, is it recommended that you go the whole nine yards and eat fully organic foods.

## A Word About Drugs

Drug allergies are not rare, and it may be wise to discontinue medications which are unnecessary.

However, certain drugs are essential and should not be stopped, such as anti-epileptics, some cardiac drugs (such as digoxin), insulin and thyroxin. Some medications, such as cortisone derivatives, need to be phased out gradually.

To be certain, it is better to discuss the implications with your doctor and ask his or her advice on stopping your treatment.

Don't be put off by the high-handedness which some doctors, sadly, are prone to when their prescriptions are questioned.

You are entitled to know the effect of any drug you are taking and precisely why you are taking it, and it may be that your doctor will not even understand the workings and side-effects of drugs being used.

The key question that you want answered is, 'Will I come to harm if I stop this drug?' Nine times out of ten the answer is, 'No'.

Don't forget, tobacco is a drug. You must stop smoking if you are serious about getting well.

Now, let's start with the easiest level diet as an entry.

## An Easy Elimination Diet (14-21 Days)

It is logical to start by eliminating only the common likely food allergies. This leaves plenty of foods to eat and you should not find this diet too onerous.

It is especially suitable for a child and consists basically of fresh meat, fish, fruit, and vegetables, with juice and water to drink.

We call it the 'Stone-Age' or 'Caveman' diet. (my first nickname with the UK press was "The Stone Age Doctor"; I used to joke this was an unfair exaggeration, I had only a few grey hairs at the time!).

## Foods you are allowed to eat:

- Any meat (not processed or smoked)

- Any vegetables (fresh or frozen, not tinned)

- Any fruit, except the citrus family (lemon etc.)

- Any fish (not processed or smoked)

- Quinoa (grain substitute)

- All fresh unsweetened fruit juices, except citrus

- Herb teas (careful: some contain citrus peel)

- Spring water, preferably bottled in glass

- Fresh whole herbs

- Salt and pepper to taste

OK, that's straightforward. There is plenty to eat, in other words. You may have to change what you usually do but you will not starve, that's for sure.

## Foods you are not allowed to eat:

- No stimulant drinks – no tea, coffee, alcohol

- No sugar, honey, additives, or sweeteners

- No grains: absolutely no wheat, corn, rye, rice, barley, oats, or millet. That means no bread, cakes, muffins, biscuits, granola, pastry, flour, or farina

- No milk or dairy produce: no skimmed milk, cream, butter, margarines, or spreads, not even goat's milk

- NO MANUFACTURED FOOD: nothing from tins, packets, bottles, or jars. If somebody labeled it, they likely added to it.

## Aspects of Elimination Dieting

Here are some important points to keep in mind:

It is vital to understand that you must not cheat on this or any other exclusion diet. This is not a slimming diet, where you can sneak a piece of chocolate cake and still lose weight.

Remember that it takes several days for food to clear your bowel and eating it as little as twice a week will prevent you clearing it from your system. If you do slip up, you will need to extend the avoidance period for several more days.

Later, when the detective work is complete, the occasional indiscretion won't matter. In the meantime, follow the instructions exactly.

Don't forget about addictions. It is quite likely that you will get withdrawal symptoms during the first few days. This is good news because it means you have given up something important. Usually the effects are mild and amount to nothing more than feeling irritable, tired, or perhaps having a headache, but be warned -it could put you in bed for a couple of days. I have seen a wheat exclusion "cold turkey" that was just as grim as narcotics.

Please also note that it is possible to be allergic even to the allowed foods - they are chosen simply because reaction to them is less common. If you are in this minority, you might even feel worse on this diet, but at least it proves you have a food allergy. In that case, try eliminating, also, the foods you are eating more of (potato is a common offender) and see if you then begin to improve.

If not, you should switch to the Eight Foods Diet, or a fast as described below.

While on the elimination diet, try to avoid hanging on to a few favorite foods and eating only those. You must eat with variety; otherwise you will risk creating reactions to the foods you are eating repeatedly.

It is senseless to go on with old habits. The whole point of exclusion dieting is to make you change what you are doing - it could be making you ill.

Don't worry about special recipes or substitutes at this stage. By the time you have fried, baked, steamed, and grilled everything once, the two weeks will almost have passed!

If in the long term it transpires that you need to keep off a food, then you can begin searching for an alternative.

Patients usually ask: What about my vitamin and mineral supplements while on an elimination diet, do I need to take those? The answer is No.

Most vitamin and mineral tablets contain hidden food ingredients, such as corn starch. Even those that say "allergy-free" formulas are misleading. They may not be made up with common allergens, such as wheat, corn, or soya derivatives; but nevertheless, vegetable ingredients are present, such as rice polishings and potato starch. To call these "allergy safe," or even hypoallergenic, is dishonest in my view.

Don't take the risk, you won't come to any harm without supplements for a short period. This leads on to another major Scott-Mumby Rule:

The biggest and commonest health hazard by far today is not what you are lacking that you should be having, but what you are already taking that you shouldn't!

In other words, giving up allergens, toxic or overload items have far more dramatic results in terms of health recovery than supplementing stuff you are deficient in.

## How Did You Get on With This Diet?

If you felt a whole lot better, skip to the section on food challenge testing:

Do not, simply because you do not improve or feel any different, make the erroneous assumption that you could not then be allergic to milk, wheat, or other banned foods.

Remember the eight nails in the shoe? This would be a serious mistake which could bar your road to recovery. You might like to try an alternative exclusion diet. Several are suggested here.

You can, in any case, carry out useful challenge tests, taking a careful note of what happens when you re-introduce a food. Careful! You do not want to hammer a pointed nail back in that shoe!

## The Eight Foods Diet (7-14 days)

Not as severe as a fast but tougher than the previous regime, is what can be called the Few Foods Diet; I prefer to use an 8-food plan. Obviously, it is more likely to succeed than the previous plan, since you are giving up more foods.

Any determined adult could cope with it, but on no account should you subject a child to this diet without his, or her, full and voluntary cooperation. It could produce a severe emotional trauma otherwise (factually, there is rarely a problem -- most children don't want to be ill and will assist you, providing they understand what you are trying to do.)

The basic idea is to produce one or two relatively safe foods for each different category we eat. Everyday foods are avoided since these include the common allergens.

Thus, we would choose fruits such as mango and papaya, not apple and banana; flesh such as duck and rabbit, not beef and pork; quail and ostrich, not chicken. The diet below contains my suggestions. You can vary it somewhat according to what is available to you locally.

**A Suggested 8-Foods Diet**

• Meat, protein: rabbit, venison

• Fowl: ostrich or quail

• Fruit: mango, kiwi fruit

• Vegetables: spinach, turnip

• Starch: buckwheat, quinoa

In addition to the stipulated foods, you are allowed salt to taste but not pepper, spring water but not herb teas or juices.

Even herbs and pepper must be challenged correctly on introduction. Note that neither of the starch foods are in the grains family. You can find out what food families are in the full volume of my book Diet Wise (details at the back of this booklet).

# Potential Problems

The main problem with such a restricted plan is boredom. However, there is enough variety here for adequate nourishment over the suggested period of seven to ten days, providing you eat a balance of all eight foods.

Exotic fruits can be expensive, but you won't need to eat them for long and, in any case, few people would deny that feeling well is worth any expense.

The chances are that, on a diet like this, you will feel well within a week, but for some conditions, such as eczema and arthritis, you will need to allow a little longer. Be prepared to go the full ten days before deciding that it isn't working.

A variation of this diet is the exotic food diet. Don't worry how many foods you can round up to eat, choose as many as you can find; just make sure they are all unusual, you personally have never eaten them, and they are not related to any common food category. You will need to learn about food families (groups of foodstuffs that are related).

## The Fast (5-7 days)

Although a fast is the ultimate approach in tracking down hidden food allergies, I don't recommend it lightly. It is quick (fast!), inexpensive, and an absolute yes-no statement on whether your illness really is caused by food allergy.

It can be tough at first, by the morning of the fifth day, you can expect to feel wonderful!

That's why fasting is popular as a religious exercise and why sometimes people with a severe attack of gastro-enteritis, who expel almost all the food content of the bowel by diarrhea and vomiting, are suddenly "cured" of some other health condition.

The real problem is that sometimes it can then be difficult to get back on to any safe foods. Everything is unmasked at once and the patient seems to react to everything he or she tries to eat. This can cause great distress.

Undertake a fast only if you are very determined or you still suspect food allergy and the other two approaches have failed.

Fasting is emphatically not suitable for certain categories of patient:

- Pregnant women

- Children

- Diabetics

- Epileptics

- Anyone seriously weakened or debilitated by chronic illness

- Anyone who has been subject to severe emotional disturbance (especially those prone to violent outbursts, or those who have tried to commit suicide)

The fast itself is simple enough—just don't eat for four or five days! You must stop smoking. Drink only bottled spring water. The whole point is to empty your bowels entirely of foodstuffs.

Thus, if you have any tendency to constipation, take Epsom salts to begin with. If in doubt, try an enema! Otherwise the effort may be wasted.

It may help to do what I call a grape-day step-down. This means eating grapes only for a day, as an easy-in step towards fasting.

Special note: A variation, which I call the 'half fast', is to eat only two foods, such as lamb and pears.

This means taking a gamble that neither lamb nor pears are allergenic, and it is not as sure-fire as the fast proper. It is permissible to carry this out for seven days, but on no account go on for longer than this.

## Food Challenge Testing

Whichever elimination approach you use, you will want to go on to testing foods, to see which are inflammatory in nature.

As soon as you feel well on an elimination regime, you can begin testing, although you must not do so before the four-day unmasking period has elapsed. Allow longer if you have been constipated.

Of course, you may never improve on an elimination diet. The problem may be something else, not a food. In that case, when three weeks (maximum) have elapsed on the simple elimination diet, two weeks on the Eight Foods Diet, or seven days on a fast, then you must begin re-introducing foods. This is vital. It is not enough to feel well on a very restricted diet; we want to know why? What are the culprits? These are the foods you must avoid long-term, not all those which are banned at the beginning.

Even if you don't feel well, as already pointed out, this does not prove you have no allergies amongst the foods you gave up. Test the foods as you re-introduce them, anyway - you may be in for a surprise

My recommended procedure is as follows, except for those coming off a fast:

1.  Eat a substantial helping of the food, preferably on its own for the first exposure. Lunch is the ideal meal for this.

2.  Choose only whole, single foods, not mixtures and recipes. Try to get supplies that have not been chemically treated in any way.

3.  Wait several hours to see if there is an immediate reaction, and if not, eat some more of it, along with a typical ordinary

evening meal.

4.  You may eat a third, or fourth, portion if you want, to be sure.

5.  Take your resting pulse (sit still for two minutes) before, and several times during the first 90 minutes after the first exposure to the food. A rise of ten or more beats in the resting pulse is a reliable sign of an allergy.

    However, no change in the pulse does not mean the food is safe, unless symptoms are absent also.

## Alkali Salts

If you do experience an unpleasant reaction, take Epsom salts. That will clear the food rapidly form your bowel.

Also, take alkali salts (a mixture of two parts sodium bicarbonate to one-part potassium bicarbonate: one teaspoonful in a few ounces of lukewarm water) should help. You can buy alkali salts on the Internet.

Discontinue further tests until symptoms have abated once more. This is very important, as you cannot properly test when symptoms are already present; you are looking for foods which trigger symptoms.

Using the above approach, you should be able to reliably test one food a day, minimum. Go rapidly if all is well, because the longer you stay off a food, the more the allergy (if there is one) will tend to die down and you may miss it.

Occasionally, patients experience a 'build up' which causes confusion and sometimes failure. Suspect this if you felt better on an exclusion diet, but you gradually became ill again when re-introducing foods, and can't really say why. Perhaps there were no noticeable reactions.

In that case, eliminate all the foods you have re-introduced until your symptoms clear again, and then re-introduce them more slowly. This time, eat the foods steadily, several times a day for three to four days before making up your mind. It is unlikely that one will slip the net with this approach.

Once you have accepted a food as safe, of course you must then stop eating it so frequently; otherwise it may become an allergy. Eat it once a day at most - only every four days when you have enough 'safe' foods to accomplish this.

## Special Instructions for Those Coming Off A Fast

Ending a fast, we do things differently. You go quicker but you must take care and DO NOT start with the obvious, tempting foods, like bread, coffee etc.

Begin only with exotic foods which you don't normally eat! *The last thing you want to happen is to get a reaction when beginning to re-introduce foods—it will mean you cannot carry on adding foods until the symptoms settle down once again.*

Instead, for the first few days, you want to build up a minimum range of 'safe' foods that you can fall back on. Papaya, rabbit, artichoke, and dogfish are the kind of thing to aim for - do the best you can with what is available according to your resources.

The other important point is that you cannot afford the luxury of bringing in one new food a day: you need to go faster than this.

When avoided even for as little as two weeks, a cyclical food allergy can die down and you may miss the proof of allergy you are looking for. It is possible to test two or even three foods a day when coming off a fast.

Pay particular attention to the pulse rate before and after each test meal and keep notes. It is important to grasp that some symptom, even if not very striking, usually occurs within the first 60 minutes when coming off a fast.

You need to be alert to this, or you will miss items and fail to improve without understanding why. If the worst happens and you are ill by the end of the day and can't say why, condemn all that day's new foods.

The buildup of foods is cumulative: that is, you start with Food A. If it is OK then the next meal is Food A + Food B, then A + B + C and so on. An example table of foods tests might be:

**Days 1- 4**
- no food

**Day 5**
- breakfast - poached salmon
- lunch - mango (plus salmon)
- dinner - steamed spinach (plus salmon and mango)

**Day 6**
- breakfast - baked pheasant, quail, or partridge + day 5
- lunch - kiwi fruit + day 5
- dinner - steamed marrow or zucchini (courgette) + day 5

**Day 7**
- breakfast -lamb chop (plus any of the above) + days 5,6
- lunch - baked potato (do not eat the skin) + days 5,6
- dinner - banana + days 5,6 etc...
- Grape not allowed on day 5, if you used a grape-day step-down

All safe foods are kept up after an allergic reaction. Therefore, if Food F causes a reaction, while you are waiting for it to clear up, you can go on eating foods A-E, until symptoms clear.

Within a few days, you should have plenty to eat, albeit monotonous. From then on, you can proceed as for those on elimination diets if you wish.

# SECTION 6:
# YOUR PERSONAL
# EXCLUSION PROGRAM

Whichever program you chose, once you have carried out the challenge tests you will have a list of items which you are intolerant of. You must now avoid these, if you are serious about your health. You have, in effect, designed your own personal diet plan for health. Use it as something you return to in times of trouble or stress, a safe platform.

There should be no rush to try and re-introduce any of these items, if at all. Design your living and eating plan without them, long-term.

However, the good news is that allergies do settle down, sometimes quite rapidly, especially if you pay attention to everything else I have explained in this book. If you develop and practice a newer safer ecological lifestyle, you may have surprisingly little further trouble.

You may feel better than you have felt in years. Many patients feel and act younger, so much so that friends and relatives often comment. I noticed this over thirty years ago and that is one of the reasons I now find myself part of the anti-aging movement.

Another Scott-Mumby maxim: a low allergy diet is the finest possible cosmetic agent for a woman's skin! She glows!

If you find your personal diet plan oppressive because you discovered quite a few reacting foods, then consider desensitization.

## Is Inflammation the Silent Killer?

It's not vitamins, growth hormone, emotional cleansing, tender loving care (TLC) or even exercise.

They all help, of course they do!

But it's pretty clear to doctors who know their stuff what the number one factor is: you need to keep inflammation to an absolute minimum.

Inflammation is an insidious disease process that goes on in all tissues and organs and greatly accelerates change and decay.

Relaxed and efficient tissues and organs perform well but when they are hot and excited, suffering from a cascade of irritating painful chemicals known as inflammatory cytokines, everything quickly starts to break down and the aging process advances rapidly.

Most of the diseases which are hallmarks of decay and aging have a strong inflammatory component. Cancer, heart disease, arthritis, arteriosclerosis, Alzheimer's disease and diabetes (yes, you read those last two right)...these are all, essentially, inflammatory diseases.

Inflammation can be caused by allergies, parasites, intolerant substances, chemical pollutants, electrical and magnetic field burdens, microbes (especially hidden chronic infections) and a host of other factors.

And inflammation is cooled down by important nutrients like omega-3 fatty acids. Now you know why they work!

## So What Can We Do?

Reduce the inflammatory load.

There is one very easy and amazingly successful way to do this, as I discovered in the late 1970s. You can do it. You don't even need a doctor to help you.

If you do it right you'll look and feel years younger within a matter of a couple of weeks. Patients I showed this to, back then, had amazing positive reactions from their friends and family: "What are you on? I want some!" and "You look ten years younger. What is your secret?"

Men looked fitter and more "present"; women looked sexier, with fewer lines and more energy, despite long hours in the kitchen or at the office.

What's the big secret?

It's eliminating stressor or inflammatory foods. These are not just allergy foods (which are very common) but other unsuitable elements in your diet.

Now this is NOT the same story as eating right for your type, the blood group diet, food combining or acid vs. alkaline foods, OR ANY OTHER DIET "THEORY".

This is about working out your own personal UNIQUE anti-inflammatory diet.

I wrote a book on how to do it for yourself. It's called Diet Wise. You can get a copy at www.DietWiseBook.com.

## Here's the Truth

The truth is that everybody is unique. That means nobody is average. That means there are an infinite number of "types". You need to dump all that stuff and grasp one simple fact: your own perfect eating plan is exclusive to you and you won't find it in anyone else's book!

You have to figure out what foods are cool for you and which ones cause an inflammatory reaction. Eat the former and avoid the latter. Your body will love it!

I can tell you how to do all this and that's the ONLY book you'll really need. I called it Diet Wise because you would truly be wise about foods, if you only learned these few very simple health principles.

Most doctors haven't a clue about nutrition. They ramble on about a "balanced" diet. By that, they seem to mean "a balance of junk", like bread, cereals, cream, tea and coffee- they don't get it and think all foods are friendly because they "feed us".

The truth is that wrong foods can cause damage; a lot of damage. The wrong foods will age you quicker than warm cookies fly out of the kitchen.

Get your full copy of Diet Wise (www.DietWiseBook.com) today and start living the anti-inflammatory life you deserve!

Here's to your enjoyable later youth!

[Shhhh! We don't mention old age round here! I'm 73 and feel like I did when I was in my 20s!]

Prof. Keith Scott-Mumby, MD, PhD

PS: Keep going for your BONUS Food Diary!

# LET YOUR BODY CHOOSE THE FOODS THAT ARE RIGHT FOR YOU!

If you have read this far and found information that is interesting and relevant to you, you will want to know more, of course...

Your own body is an ideal medical officer! It knows what suits you and what doesn't. You just have to "consult" it in the right way.

Dr. Keith Scott-Mumby's masterwork, Diet Wise (312 pages), tells you step by step how to work out which foods are safe FOR YOU and which foods inflame your tissues.

Remember: inflammation is at the core of almost all diseases and even aging itself. You do not want inflammation in your body. Everyone is different in which foods they react to. You must not trust stories about other people's "safe foods" or "super-foods" which worked. It will probably not be relevant for you.

What Dr. Keith has brought to the world is a marvellous and effective system for creating your own, PERSONAL, ideal diet. It's not like anyone else's!

It's an exploration everyone should undertake at least once in a lifetime. Your reward for doing so is abundant health and vitality, plus a lot more years of active life.

Read more about this amazing book here:
**www.DietWiseBook.com**

**Also, see the final pages of this booklet for exciting stories from those who took the trouble to work out their own "safe diet".**

# DIET WISE

## TOXIC FOODS ARE COMMON AND CAUSE A LOT OF HARM.
## EVERYONE IS DIFFERENT. FIND OUT YOURS

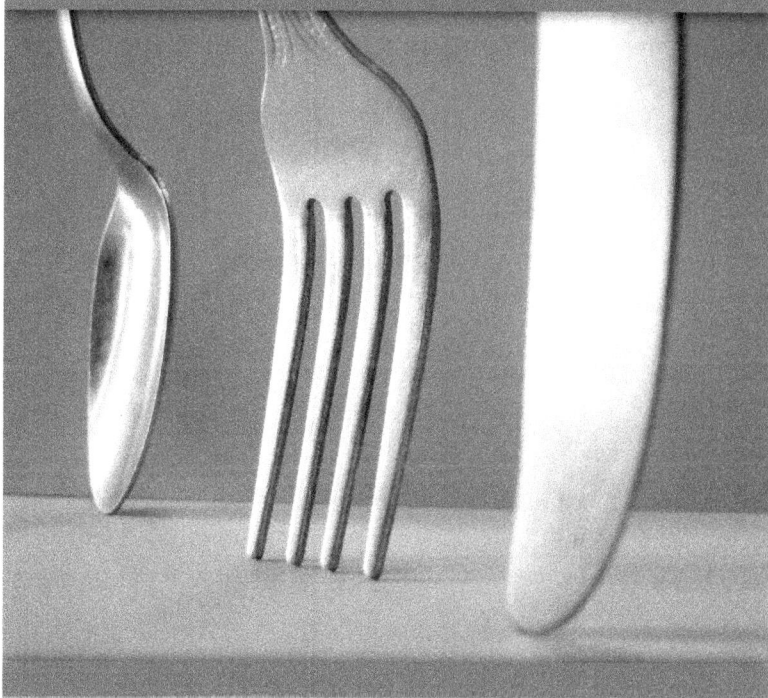

### BY
### PROF. KEITH SCOTT-MUMBY MB ChB, MD, PhD

*This is the doctor who changed the face of medicine in Britain. They call him the "Number One Allergy Detective". Now he's here in the US.*

# BONUS: 12-WEEK FOOD SYMPTOM DIARY

It is a good idea to keep a food diary during your experiments with food. Write down everything you eat at each meal, or between meals, and mark in any symptoms which you experience, with the time of onset in relation to meals.

It is often possible to spot a pattern which recurs time and time again, but which is not evident when relying only on short-term memory.

Warning: a food diary does tend to make you very conscious of food, which is probably a good thing in the short term. However, taking the long view, try to avoid the exercise making you too introverted about feelings and symptoms, otherwise it can start becoming an obsession.

Many allergy patients become so consumed by anxiety about what they are eating that they cannot eat or socialize normally.

Food allergy investigations, as described here, are merely a tool not an end and should not become a way of life, otherwise family and friends will feel excluded and that in turn leads to rejection.

Many "amateur" gung-ho food allergy books tend to create this major social incompetence, because the authors do not have sufficient experience to be aware of the dangers (and likely because they too are obsessive).

Make no mistake, food allergy restrictions can ruin relationships and break up marriages, if it is taken to extreme, as many know to their cost. I do not automatically take the patient's side but sympathize with both points of view (because ultimately, I see this as in the patient's broader interests).

Eating can become a psychological burden on the patient and intolerable nuisance to family and friends, if you go too far. True health does not mean isolation from society, it means full social wellbeing included in the deal.

The food diary is merely a tool and should be discontinued as soon as practicable.

I've included a simplistic 12-week food diary for you to use to track the foods, drinks, medications, or activities that cause an adverse reaction to you.

## My Food Symptom Diary: Day 1

| Time of day | Foodstuffs<br>Be sure to list actual<br>ingredients, not just "muffin" | Symptoms<br>Time when started is crucial |
| --- | --- | --- |
| | | |

## My Food Symptom Diary: Day 2

| Time of day | Foodstuffs<br>Be sure to list actual ingredients, not just "muffin" | Symptoms<br>Time when started is crucial |
|---|---|---|
| | | |

## My Food Symptom Diary: Day 3

| Time of day | Foodstuffs<br>Be sure to list actual<br>ingredients, not just "muffin" | Symptoms<br>Time when started is crucial |
|---|---|---|
| | | |

# My Food Symptom Diary: Day 4

| Time of day | Foodstuffs Be sure to list actual ingredients, not just "muffin" | Symptoms Time when started is crucial |
| --- | --- | --- |
| | | |

## My Food Symptom Diary: Day 5

| Time of day | Foodstuffs<br>Be sure to list actual<br>ingredients, not just "muffin" | Symptoms<br>Time when started is crucial |
|---|---|---|
| | | |

# My Food Symptom Diary: Day 6

| Time of day | Foodstuffs<br>Be sure to list actual<br>ingredients, not just "muffin" | Symptoms<br>Time when started is crucial |
|---|---|---|
| | | |

# My Food Symptom Diary: Day 7

| Time of day | Foodstuffs<br>Be sure to list actual<br>ingredients, not just "muffin" | Symptoms<br>Time when started is crucial |
| --- | --- | --- |
| | | |

# My Food Symptom Diary: Day 8

| Time of day | Foodstuffs Be sure to list actual ingredients, not just "muffin" | Symptoms Time when started is crucial |
|---|---|---|
| | | |

## My Food Symptom Diary: Day 9

| Time of day | Foodstuffs<br>Be sure to list actual<br>ingredients, not just "muffin" | Symptoms<br>Time when started is crucial |
|---|---|---|
| | | |

# My Food Symptom Diary: Day 10

| Time of day | Foodstuffs<br>Be sure to list actual<br>ingredients, not just "muffin" | Symptoms<br>Time when started is crucial |
|---|---|---|
| | | |

# DIET WISE BOOK TESTIMONIALS

"Diet Wise was a breakthrough for me. I had wondered if I had food allergies besides what I already knew (shellfish), and so I gave the elimination diet a try. Longest 5 days of my life, but very revealing. I eliminated everything he said to, plus I also eliminated potatoes because I was suspecting them as a problem. While on the diet, I ate a container of cashews, and the next morning I awoke to a puffed up left eye. Clearly, I was also allergic to cashews. Now those are eliminated! Also, strawberries gave me a rash on my hands, so I didn't realize I was intolerant of those, too.

After adding back foods one at a time, I look and feel better than ever. I think you can follow Paleo, Atkins, whatever popular diet today and not get the results you want because you are intolerant to foods that most people aren't. This uncovers what YOU can and can't tolerate. It's a good read, good logic behind it. Definitely made me think about some foods I overeat, and I am encouraged to do more food rotating, perhaps consider seasonal foods more."

-       J.U., USA

"Diet Wise literally changed my life! I was so ill last winter, (2014) prescribed inhalers, told I'd need to go on oxygen, told I had asthma, COPD, pneumonia, echo cardiograms, CAT scans ... I'd feel better for awhile and then I'd be sick again. I started following the suggestions in this book about eliminating foods to see what I might be allergic/intolerant to ... and incredibly – within a few short weeks, I was well and have been well ever since. I am now able to occasionally eat a loved food, but as long as I stay away from my intolerance foods, I feel like a million dollars. Start slipping some of the foods back into my diet and immediately begin with burning eyes, nasal congestion, wheezing and I don't hang around long enough to find out how bad it might get. I am hopeful this coming winter will not be a repeat of last year.

As a personal opinion, Dr. Keith is a bit of arrogance and a whole bunch of down-to-earth truth rolled together into a likeable guy. Don't always agree with his take on certain views, but am open enough to recognize that he's onto something and that he has certainly helped restore my health and life. I get a kick out of him. Hope this helps someone out there."

-      L.B., USA

"Diet Wise is an excellent book and the concepts are essential for anyone with health problems. All foods have chemicals in then naturally that some people cannot metabolize. These can cause anything from mild to horrifying symptoms. When I was a child I had horrible stomach aches. I went through various medical tortures including an appendectomy with no benefit. Eventually I figured out that this was caused by eating spicy foods like pepper, garlic, onions and other vegetables considered healthy.

As an adult I started having most of the symptoms of multiple sclerosis. This included numb hands, barbershop syndrome and extreme difficulty standing and walking. It was much worse on Saturdays and I wondered if going out to eat on Friday nights was causing my problem. I figured out that the corn oil in the restaurant food was the villain and my symptoms went away. Later I found a book reporting that about 70% of MS is greatly improved by removing improper oils from the diet.

These are just two examples from my life. This book explains the problem and how to find out what foods might be problems for you. Removing the foods that poison you may be the most important health factor. Even more important than removing processed foods, eating healthy foods, exercise, posture, fresh air, sunshine or any of the other very important health principles.

Having this information is vital to people with health problems."

-       John F Kilpatrick

"Many diet books tell you their method is customized for you. They're all wrong. Diet Wise is truly a program made for each individual person. It's like a second chance in life to learn what good and bad foods are for my body specifically. The other great thing is that there's a huge selection of foods to eat during the initial program that will figure out what foods cause problems. I've been dieting pretty much all my life and have tried a lot of programs. This is a great one. Dr. Scott-Mumby presents a lot of medical information, but it was very understandable. This program is really unique, and I'd recommend it to everyone."

-       S.L. Bartlett

Don't forget to get your FULL COPY of my book **Diet Wise** so you can take all the things you've learned here to the next level!

You can find it at **www.DietWiseBook.com!**

To your good health!

Prof. Keith

www.ingramcontent.com/pod-product-compliance
Lightning Source LLC
Chambersburg PA
CBHW060643280326
41933CB00012B/2130